NUTRITION EDUCATION: AN IMPORTANT PILLAR OF HEALTH

NUTRITION EDUCATION: AN IMPORTANT PILLAR OF HEALTH

Dr. Khushboo Gupta

HEMAKSHEE PUBLICATION

Nutrition Education: An Important Pillar of Health

Author: Dr. Khushboo Gupta

ISBN: 978-81-969920-8-8

Publisher: Hemakshee Publication

Publication Year: 2024

CONTENTS

PREFACE

Nutrition is a science that deals with the study of nutrients in food, how the body utilizes them as well the relationship between diet, health and disease. Proper and optimum nutrient intake via food can provide therapeutic benefits also. Nutrition science not only deals with the quantity and quality of nutrients but also tells us about different food allergies and knowledge regarding nutrient content of any food item that can be affected by different processing and preservation techniques used to prepare that particular food item. The in-depth knowledge of food, nutrition and health can be gained through various graduate and post graduate courses.

As nutrition is a health concerned topic and it is a dire need to spread knowledge of nutrition among common people to upgrade their living status and quality of life. This can be easily done by using nutrition education techniques to the masses.

Nutrition education is a continuing process of teaching the science of nutrition to a person or a group. Health professionals specially nutritionists, dietitians, subject matter specialists and master trainers have different roles in educating people in different settings, i.e., individual, in the clinic, in community or in long term health care facility. The main focus of nutrition education is to develop permanent healthy behavioral changes in the person. Due to various reasons common people don't have access of healthy food and optimum nutrient consumption, thus, in India very first time 'nutrition week' is celebrated in September, 1982 when the Government of India began a drive to inform the people of country and also motivate them to live long and healthy life. Our Prime Minister 'Shri Narendra ji Modi' shows special interest in nutritional upliftment of the society. As our Ayurveda and ancient Indian culture depict that "one's food can be another person's poison". Thus proper knowledge and awareness of different components of food and nutrition is very essential for maintaining good quality of life.

Keeping this point of view "Jeevan Asheesh Sameeti", a non-profit organization from Kota city, Rajasthan and YouTube Channel "Dietitian Ki Salah" (an educational plateform for integrated health, wholesome nutrition, fitness and food) celebrated 'National Nutrition Month' in September, 2022 and organize an essay writing competition for masses on various topics related to nutrition and health. People participate in this activity enthusiastically and appreciate the joint efforts of "Jeevan Asheesh Sameeti" and YouTube Channel "Dietitian Ki Salah" for this endeavour. Main aim of this activity was to aware common people about uses of numerous healthy aspects of nutrition in daily life, therefore, we are compiling all those essays in the form of an edited book.

The edited book volume is primarily intended to be a collection of short chapters written by research scholars, academicians and faculty members of their respective fields. Chapters of this book entitled **"Nutrition Education: An Important Pillar of Health"** particularly based on different topics of nutrition science, i.e., importance of nutrition in daily life, flavours of Bengal, flavours of Ramadan, Indian spices, celebrate a world of flavours, nutrition in bed bound patients, why nutrition is essential and importance of homemade pickles in daily diet.

I envisage the book to serve as a reference book for common people. This book will be very useful for students all over in India and Abroad, academicians, public health specialists, community science specialists, community development professionals, programmers of national and international agencies, and people of grassroot level to aware them about different issues pertaining to nutrition as well as libraries of relevant collages and institutions.

This is my seventh book in the series of community upliftment. The first book titled as "Vridhopayogi Vyanjan: Vridhjano ke liye Upcharatmak Pak Vidhiyan (year 2016)" which contains more than 65 healthy food recipes developed, prepared and clinically verified by myself alone, tailored with the nutritional needs of the geriatric population.

Second book titled as "Community Science and Sustainable Community Development (Year 2021)" that provides excellent research data related to different aspects of community which will be helpful to strengthen the sustainability of a community in terms of health, nutrition, wellness and economy.

My next three books are the three distinct volumes of title "75 years of Indian Independence: Food and Nutritional Achievements, Opportunities and Challenges (Year 2022)" that provide enriched research data pertaining to various aspects of health, lifestyle, tourism, agriculture, antenatal or post natal diet, nutritional status, cognition and nutrition, etc., that will be extremely helpful to improve quality of life of the individuals ultimately making healthy and sustainable community.

My sixth book entitled "Aazadi ka Amrit Mahotsav: Community Science Achievements, Opportunities and Challenges" particularly based on different disciplines of community science, i.e., food science and nutrition, food security, advancement in food preservation and processing, sustainable breeding and cultivation approaches in agriculture, importance of prebiotics, role of therapeutic diet, importance of nutrition for pregnant ladies and children, how cognitive development is affected by nutritional status of the children, spiritual development, skill based learning system DEASA, effect of social media on community development.

With great pleasure, I would like to extend my sincere thanks to all the authors of the chapters for reporting their thoughts and experience related to their research and also for patiently addressing reviewer's comments and diligently adhering hectic deadlines to have the book published in timely manner. Their constant support and cooperation has made my task as editor a pleasure. I believe that this book is an important contribution to the community in addressing research work from numerous domains of community science.

It is my sincere hope that many more will join us in this time-critical endeavour and this book will stimulate discussions and generate helpful comments to improve future projects.

Happy reading and feedback awaited.

Dr. Khushboo Gupta
Assistant Professor
Trilok Singh TT College,
Lakshmangarh, Sikar,
Rajasthan, India

ACKNOWLEDGEMENTS

It is indeed a great pleasure for me to express my profound gratitude to these eminent yet approachable personalities who helped me to bring this humble endeavour to its fruitful completion.

I am grateful to almighty God, who provided me an opportunity and ability to accomplish the great task, who in every moment of my life, always blessed me beyond my imagination, helped me in every difficult time and gave me strength and perseverance. Whatever I am today is just because of them.

I deeply recognize the efforts by all authors for their contribution without whom this book will not look like what it is today. They deserve a special round of applause.

Finally, I acknowledge the sincere efforts of my family which has been the nucleus around which all my efforts have crystallized. No one can conquer without a strong base. I bow my head with great respect to my grandparents and hope that this work makes you proud. Thanks for your blessings. Words would fail to express my heartfelt veneration and deep sense of admiration to my loving siblings Er. Surbhee Gupta and Er. Saurabh Gupta for their love, affection, moral support, encouragement and help in every possible way to complete my work. Their unwavering faith in me has always been a source of constant inspiration for me.

I express deep and heartfelt obligation to my parents Mrs. Archana Gupta and Dr. Lok Mani Gupta for their patience, cordial affection, will power, blessings, moral support and for being my driving force. Their love provided inspiration and motivation, without which this work would not have been completed. They are the real architects of my life. They inspired me to build castles when all I had was a fistful of sand. They always stood by me during all thick and thin. Without their support, patience, sacrifice, forebearance and unalloyed love, this work would never have seen the light of the day.

I want to express feelings of utmost gratitude towards my parents-in-laws for their blessings. I owe Heartfelt thanks to a very special person my husband CA Dinesh Agrawal for being there for me at every step of this writing journey. My husband's good spirits, patience, constant support and encouragement made it possible to accomplish this task. I appreciate my kids, Hemakshee Agrawal and Devansh Agrawal for abiding my ignorance and the patience they showed during this endeavour. Their cute smile inspired me to go forward and their playful and naughty activities relaxed me during my tough times. Words would never say how grateful I am to both of you.

In the end, I want to express my sincere and deepest gratitude to everyone who, in their own way, directly or indirectly, have helped me to complete this book but could not have found separate names, so just in case: thank you to whom it may concern.

Dr. Khushboo Gupta

Ph.D. (Food and Nutrition)

EDITOR BIOGRAPHY

Dr. Khushboo Gupta is a PhD Home Science (Food Science and Nutrition) from Banasthali Vidyapith, Newai, India. She has been teaching subject including food chemistry, food analysis, therapeutic nutrition, human nutrition, human physiology and community nutrition, etc. Presently she is working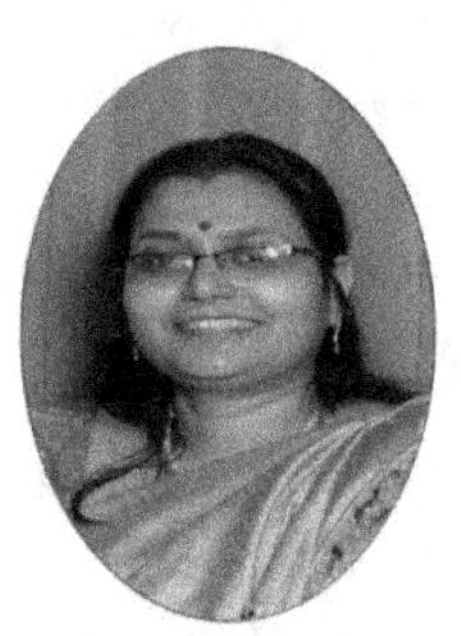 as Assistant Professor in Trilok Singh TT College, Laxmangarh, Sikar, Rajasthan.

She is MSc Gold medalist and had cleared UGC-NET and RPSC-SET examination. Dr Gupta holds Advance Diploma in French Language from Banasthali Vidyapith; Diploma in Naturopathy and Yoga (NDDY) from Gandhi Smarak Prakritik Chikitsa Samiti (Regd.), New Delhi; Certificate in Homeopathic Medicinal System conducted by Vardhman Mahaveer Open University, Kota and Certificate in Statistical Techniques and Applications. She has featured in several programs of All India Radio and Radio Banasthali (FM 90.4).

Dr. Khushboo is actively involved in community activities especially those concerned with self-employment, health and wellness, optimum nutrition and how to improve quality of life of a person and family. She is the keynote speaker and founder of her YouTube channel "Dietitian Ki Salah" through which she provides education related to optimum health, wellness and nutrition to masses. Dr. Gupta has published about more than 30 research papers in reputed national and international journals; 5 book chapters in five different edited books, several news paper and magazine articles related to health, nutrition and new food product formulation. She authored one book related to elderly nutrition; edited two books related to community science and three books (edited books) related to food science for upliftment of the individuals of the society. She presented her research work in more than 25 national and international conferences. Her research is primarily in the area of food processing entrepreneurial skill Inculcation and geriatric nutrition and her research on food formulation using RSM has culminated into the successful filing of a patent that has been published.

In past she had worked as Assistant Professor (Food and Nutrition) in Modi University, Laxmangarh, Sikar; worked as Master Trainer in Agriculture University, Kota. During her PhD she had worked as UGC- SRF in Banasthali Vidyapith, Newai. One feather in her cap is that she had worked as regular trainee dietitian in dietetics department of Post Graduate Institute of Medical Education and Research (PGIMER), Chandigarh and got her short-term attachment certificate. She won many awards in different seminars and conferences for her contribution in scientific world. Apart from them, she is rewarded with Teacher Honour award by Lions Club Kota South (September, 2017) and 'Award of Honour' given by All Rajasthan Qualified Homoeopathic Doctors Association in Homoeopathic Scientific Seminar, 2017

She is the life member of many reputed institutes i.e. Nutrition Society of India, Indian Dietetic Association, The Indian Science Congress Association and Institute of Scholars and giving her services for upliftment of community.

LIST OF CONTRIBUTORS

1. **Shivani Gupta**, (Msc, UGC NET), Multani Mal Modi College, Patiala, India

2. **Dr. Purrvi Patel**, Homoeopathic physician, nutritionist, Mindfulness coach for adults and teens, Author.

3. **Dr. Shweta Habbu Acharya**, Reader, Dept. of Public Health Dentistry, Dr. HSRSM Dental College and Hospital, Hingoli

4. **Dr. Lok Mani Gupta**, Homoeopathic Doctor, Secretary, Jeevan Asheesh Sameeti (A non profit organization), Kota Rajasthan

5. **Mrs. Archana Gupta**, Homemaker, Kota, Rajasthan

6. **Dr Aamena Zaidi**, Assistant Professor , Department of Human Nutrition School of health Sciences, Chhatrapati Shahuji Maharaj University, Kanpur

7. **Dr Shivangi Gupta**, (PhD Home Science), Working as Clinical Dietician, Chandigarh

8. **Taskeen Fatima**, Assistant Professor, St. Joseph's College for Women, Civil Lines , Gorakhpur

9. **Aishwarya Das**, Research scholar, Department of Home Science Mahila Mahavidyalaya, Banaras Hindu University, Varanasi

10. **Dr. Devdatta Lad**, Department of Zoology Wilson College Chowpatty, Mumbai 400 007

11. **Neelam**, Research scholar, Department of Home Science Mahila Mahavidyalaya, Banaras Hindu University, Varanas

12. **Ranjana Sinha**, Research Scholar, P.G. Department of Home Science, Magadh University, Bodhgaya

13. **Tanushri Vijay**, Research Scholars, Department of Human/Child Development, Mohanlal Sukhadia University, Udaipur, Rajasthan

If readers have any query related to any chapter of the book, kindly contact with the corresponding author of the chapter. Authors of the chapters are solely responsible for their work.

1

WHY NUTRITION IS ESSENTIAL??

Dr. Lok Mani Gupta

Homoeopathic Doctor

Secretary, Jeevan Ashish Samitee

Nutrition is very important for every living creature in universe be it nature or human being. Apart from human being, grass, shrubs, trees, crops, birds, animals all need proper food and nutrition to develop and flourish. Nutrition is needed from womb to tomb for each and every creature to have a normal healthy growth physically as well as mentally. Here we will talk about nutrition for human being.

One of the four legs of table for health is proper nutrition which is most neglected now-a-days. People are eating food for taste or just to follow others without knowing their benefits. Balanced healthy diet is needed to remain healthy. It plays very important role to develop and maintain healthy mental status also.

Healthy diet including the required values of nutrients like carbohydrates, proteins, fats, vitamins, minerals and water depending on age and sex, affects the germinative factor of both. It is essential for healthy development of ova and sperms which are responsible for healthy and timely fertilization for a couple.

Healthy diet is very important for pregnant mother as she has to feed two lives, one herself and another foetus, taking growth and shape in her womb, where additional intake of macro as well as micro nutrients is very essential for ethical developments .

To Understand the importance of micro nutrients, we must remember the importance of pinch of salt in heap of flour which is enough to make the food taste better hence we must not neglect the importance of proper supplement of requisite nutritive diet which is very essential to germinate and cultivate the three healthy layer of early foetus to develop and take the proper shape.

Consumption of inappropriate diet during three trimesters of pregnancy can cause various malformations in the foetus as well as it can cause less deposition of nutrients in the mothers that is required after delivery (during breast feeding) for growth and development of the baby. Contrarily, if recommended dietary amount of macro and micronutrients were given to the lady during her pregnancy, innumerous cases of infertility, miscarriage and mal developments can be treated with proper dietary changes only.

Apart from normal developments proper intake of food and nutrition builds a person strong euough to face various antizen antibody reactions by increasing the immunity which was much hyped and discussed during the COVID era. Vitamin C was prescribed all over the world for immunity boost.

Our government has understood it very well and is running various motivational schemes to provide the healthy dietary support to pregnant woman and child. Some schemes are as follows

1 Latest scheme is to provide nutrition kits to every pregnant lady for fulfillment of daily need of macro and micro nutrients in diet.

2 Motivating NGO'S to distribute healthy diet kils to pregnant ladies.

3 Bal Poshahar scheme

4 Mother and child care programs.

5 School mid day meal program.

2

HOMEMADE PICKLES: WAREHOUSE OF PROBIOTICS AND ANTIOXIDANT

Mrs. Archana Gupta

Homemaker, Kota

Probiotics are the healthy bacterias that reside in the get and are needed for healthy functioning of human gut. Mostly people know some milk sources that provide probiotics in human diet. In this article you will get to know a new food item that has rich probiotic content and easily available in every Indian households.

Summer season in india is not only known for refreshing local cold drinks like sharbat, chhach, lassi, thandai, panna but also known for zesty homemade pickles or achaar. They are treasured age old condiments whipped up in summers of every year. Traditional home made pickles could be an important player in ensuring food quality, food safety as well as they could be worked as a source of micronutrients and antioxidants.

Now a days modern Indians avoid to eat pickles as they consider it bad food item due to its high salt content. But its not true as the traditional pickles are not only made with salt only but preparation process includes fruits/vegetables, sugars/salt, spices and herbs and oils many pickles are made up with fermentation process, that creats gal microflora in it which prevent the food spoilage and enhance the shelf life of pickles. Fermented pickles have unique flavor change in textual properties and digestibility of food certain micronutrients are produced i.e.

Riboflavin, folate, cobalamin , thiamine in the course of fermentation apart from that these fermented pickles are the warehouse of nutritious bioactive compounds and antioxidant (phenols flavonoids and sterols) that can be helpful to meet the hidden hunger.

Many research studies have shown that the fermented pickles (from furits)/vegetables/fish/meat) olds a probiotics culture of 10^6- 10^7 CFU/g , therefore these pickles have potential therapeutic benefits over certain problems like, gastritis, diabetes, hyper cholesterolemia they show anti-infectious anti-tumor , anti-inflammatory and anti-mutagenic activity. Pickles are the integral part of indian diet (either in nort or south) from many centuries and its combilion goes well with almost every indian food.

After reading this article you can understand why our food is best because not only it taste good but small moderate amount of pickle consumption has multiple scientifically proven health benefits.

Pickles are fermented using two methods.

1. Sweet fermented pickles are prescribed by a combination of sugar, spices, fruits/vegetables and lactin or acitic active acid.

2. Sour fermented pickles are prepared by using 2-5% salt solution in 1-2 week period natural occurring bacterias develop in the food and produce lactic acid that consequently prevents the growth of spoilage causing bacteria in food.

3

CELEBRATE A WORLD OF FLAVOURS

Shivani Gupta

(MSc, UGC-NET)

Department of Foods and Nutrition, Multani Mal Modi College, Patiala

Just like you celebrate different festivals in every corner of the world. It's time to celebrate the various flavors that are present everywhere, but you are not conscious of it. It's time to embrace the diversity that exists in your food. It's time to appreciate the so-called little things, but in reality, they are very essential to your lives. It's time to worship your "Annapurna". It's time to express gratitude for the food you eat. **It's time to celebrate a world of flavors.**

Food is the basic requirement of an individual, everyone needs it, and it connects you all in a variety of flavors, textures, colors, tastes, aromas, and many more. India has a rich bank of flavors, look at various regional cuisine like northern cuisine, western cuisine, southern cuisine, and eastern cuisines, street foods, meals, thalis, starters, appetizers, mains, desserts, snacks, enriched with various flavors with the help of various ingredients like asafoetida, bay leaves, cardamom, cinnamon, cloves, coconut, fennel seeds, fenugreek, peppercorns, dried mango powder, curry leaves, banana leaves, cumin, mustard seeds, garam masala, garlic, ginger, saffron, rose water, tamarind, turmeric, mint, coriander, etc.

But now the question arises. **How you can celebrate this occasion?** You can celebrate this occasion in many ways such as exploring different cuisines, trying different dishes around the world, adding different herbs and spices, experimenting with innovative and unique recipes, and discussing your cultural foods among your friends, family, and your social environment.

While exploring different flavors, you get to know about other's cultural foods, their rituals, and their way of living, and then you can easily connect with their social environment which brings harmony, peace, love, joy, and integrity to the world. It helps to build rapport between individuals. It helps to reduce conflicts, arguments, disputes, and differences as it enables you to understand others' ways of living, and the perspectives of others. It helps you to build a sense of respect for other's cultures, too.

It also helps in practicing dietary diversification which means the availability of various nutrients in your body which meets your various nutrient requirements of the body, keeps you away from various micronutrient deficiencies and also automatically promotes holistic development of an individual. The development of the individual means the development of the nation. It also shows the positive outcomes in mental illness and stress and also reduces the feeling of loneliness as one can share their problems with trustworthy people and also find ways to deal with them.

There is a popular saying, **"The way to a person's heart is through the stomach"**. If you want to understand another culture or person, try their cultural food. This is a very good start to initiate a deep, meaningful, and long-lasting relationship. Relationships that start with sharing food blossom well.

Together we are strength. To combat various diseases, deficiencies, malnutrition, and nutritional challenges you all have to come together and should work as a team. Every individual has to take responsibility not only for lifting himself but also for the upliftment of the society.

4

IMMUNITY BOOSTER FOODS

Dr Aamena Zaidi

Assistant Professor

Department of Human Nutrition

School of Health Sciences

Chhatrapati Shahuji Maharaj University, Kanpur

Evidence from a variety of fruits, vegetables, roots, spices, and herbs suggests that numerous nutritional supplements can improve immune function, hence lowering the risk of several illnesses. As a result, using natural substances may offer an alternative to traditional preventative and therapeutic measures.

The following are some of the nutrients' health benefits:

1. Zinc

It is cofactor in numerous biological processes. It controls inflammatory activity and performs antioxidant and antiviral functions. 35% decrease in the frequency of acute respiratory infections is shown with oral Zn supplementation. Due to its antiviral, anti-inflammatory, and antioxidant properties, zinc is thought to be a viable supportive treatment for infection.

Sources: Oysters, red meat, poultry, beans, nuts, crab, lobster, whole grains, breakfast cereals, and dairy products.

2. Vitamin D

It is essential for immune modulation, antioxidant protection, and antiviral defence. Vitamin D insufficiency increases susceptibility to acute viral respiratory infections, while its supplementation enhances immuneresponses.

Sources: Sunlight. Food sources include Salmon, Herring fish, cod liver oil, Egg yolk, Mushrooms and Vitamin D fortified foods

3. Vitamin C

Because it is important for immune function, Vitamin C is able to prevent illness. It also enhances capacity to fight infection. Upper respiratory illnesses, such as the common cold, can be less severe when supplemented with Vitamin C. It is a strong antioxidant. Therefore, Vitamin C can aid with reducing symptoms, boosting the immune system, and preventing infection by having an anti-inflammatory and antioxidant effect.

Sources: Citrus fruits

4. Curcumin

Antibacterial, antiviral, antifungal, antioxidant, and anti-inflammatory activity are the biological effects of curcumin. It has a anti-viral impact on human papillomavirus, human immunodeficiency virus, herpes simplex virus type 2 and Zika virus. It works to prevent the spread of viruses by preventing viral entrance into cells, preventing viral protease encapsulation, preventing viral reproduction, and modifying a number of signalling pathways.

Sources: Turmeric

5. Cinnamaldehyde

A well-known dietary phytonutrient renowned for its anti-inflammatory effects is cinnamonaldehyde which is widely distributed in the cinnamon essential oils. Cinnamon's flavour and odour are primarily derived from its trans-isomer form, which is where it predominates.

Sources: Cinnamon

6. Allicin

A well-known plant or herb noted for its many nutritional benefits, garlic is a member of the Allium (onion) family. Due to its anti-inflammatory, antioxidant, and antiviral characteristics, allicin, the main thiosulfinate found in fresh garlic extract, has demonstrated a number of health advantages. Ajoene, allicin, allyl, methyl thiosulfinate, and methyl allyl thiosulfinate are some of the chemicals in garlic that have viricidal properties.

Sources: Garlic

7. Piperine

Black pepper has a long history of use in many different cuisines and is one of the most important medicinal plants. Piperine is obtained from ethanolic extract of black pepper. Piperine has potent anti-inflammatory properties. By encouraging phagocytes to engage in phagocytic activity, piperine supports innate immunity. Additionally, piperine is a strong antioxidant that guards against oxidative damage by disarming free radicals.

Sources: Black pepper

8. Selenium

Common foods including corn, garlic, onion, cabbage, and broccoli are high in selenium. It is a necessary micronutrient that has a significant impact on the immune system as well as several physiological functions. Through incorporation into seleno-proteins in the body, selenium has a biological impact. Selenium boosts immunity through its non-enzymatic activity as a cofactor for enzymes involved in essential post-translational modifications of proteins.

Sources: Sea foods, organ meats, muscle meats, cereals and dairy products.

9. Propolis

Honeybees manufacture a substance called propolis that is known to have a variety of biological qualities, such as anti-microbial, anti-inflammatory, dermato-protective, laxative, anti-diabetic, anti-tumor, and immunomodulatory action. Additionally, elements in honey propolis inhibit a number of viruses, including influenza A1 virus, herpes simplex, human cytomegalovirus, and dengue virus type 2.

Sources: Resinous mixture, made by the honeybees from substances collected from tree or other plant buds, plant exudates, or resins found in the stem, branches, or leaves of different plants.

10. Probiotics

The commonly used probiotics are Bifidobacterium and Lactobacillus species, followed by the Streptococcus, Enterococcus, Bacillus, and Escherichia coli. Probiotics not only support the health of the gut but also improves system functioning and regulation. Consumption of Bifidobacterium and Lactobacillus have found to help in clearing the influenza virus in the respiratory tract. In general, probiotics exert anti-inflammatory and immunomodulatory effects.

Sources: Yoghurt

11. Lactoferrin

A naturally occurring, non-toxic glycoprotein known as lactoferrinhas been tested against a variety of viruses. It is essential for blocking the entry and reproduction of the virus. Studies have demonstrated that it has immunomodulatory and antioxidant effects by causing T-cell activation and reducing interleukin levels. In infant's formula, it is mostly utilised as a nutritional supplement.

Sources

Cow milk, Human milk and Colostrum

12. Quercetin

A well-known antioxidant with anti-inflammatory and antiviral properties is quercetin. It prevents viral cell fusion and virus invasion. Quercetin and Vitamin C together have been demonstrated to have synergistic antiviral and immunomodulatory effects in other investigations as well.

Sources: Apples, honey, cherries, citrus fruits, and green leafy vegetables.

5

SPORTS NUTRITION-FUELING YOUR BODY THE RIGHT WAY

Tanu Shri Vijay

Research Scholars,

Department of Human/Child Development,

Mohanlal Sukhadia University, Udaipur, Rajasthan

Sports are an intense physical activity that requires proper nourishment. Nutrition is the process of supplying one's body with enough food to maintain its health and keep it functioning properly. Sports nutrition is essential for all athletes. Sports nutrition encompasses the process of planning and cooking meals that a person can consume while participating in a sport. It is used to help with weight control, performance, and general health. Choosing the right nutritional plan can help an athlete perform better and stay healthy during their sport participation.

Sports nutrition plans include food sources, quantities, timing, and types of food for athletes to consume. It helps athletes train and work on their diet plans during training sessions and competitions. It also supports athletes during periods of sickness or fatigue. Many factors go into the development of a sports nutrition plan, including age, gender, weight, height and previous sports experience. The food recommendations will be different for each athlete depending on his physical condition. For example, if an athlete has injuries, weak spots or fatigue, he/she will need to supplement their plan with extra protein and carbohydrates to support their needs. Various sports need different nutritional plans due to the amount of physical activity they require. For example, running events require high carbohydrate intake during the competition due to the high intensity of the exercise. Other sports benefit from eating lots of protein such as weightlifting or bodybuilding competitions. Meals should be well-balanced including plenty of carbohydrate, protein, fat and vitamins and minerals. Additionally, it should include specific meal timings that the athlete must adhere to during his training hours or competitions. Failure to do so may cause fatigue and slow down performance- which could lead to injuries or deaths in extreme cases.

How competitive events affect the sports nutrition plans depends on how long they last. Short-duration competitive events require athletes to eat more carbohydrates than normal due to their limited time frame. Most events last less than twelve hours; however, extreme sports competitions can last several days or even weeks. During this time, athletes have little time to eat so they can replenish their energy levels with food sources rich in protein and fat. Failure to do so could seriously deplete an athlete's energy levels over time, causing serious fatigue and possibly leading to death by heat stroke or starvation.

It is significant to remember that athletes need a healthy diet in order to compete at their best. Diet has a huge impact on training, and a healthy diet helps an athlete stay consistent during challenging sessions. Athletes who eat foods containing the appropriate balance of nutrients will stay healthy and perform at their peak. Salmon is one of the foods that is recommended for athletes because it contains omega-3 fatty acids and proteins, which can aid to reduce inflammation and improve athletic performance. According to research, athletes who had seafood twice a week in amounts of roughly 8 ounces benefited from its anti-inflammatory properties. Berries are another illustration; according to a study, athletes should select the berries with the deepest colour to guarantee they are consuming a variety of antioxidants that help prevent the formation of free radicals in the body during exercise. A 2009 study found that consuming lots of antioxidants helps maintain strength and muscle (MacMillan). A good nutritional plan helps the athletes stay healthy and build muscle during their sports practice or competition. The athletes should establish dietary routines that allow them to consume the recommended amounts of carbs, proteins, vitamins, and minerals. Athletes should hydrate adequately. Every vitamin is essential for maximising an athlete's performance. Due to insufficient energy, muscular injury, and dehydration, an imbalanced diet and poor fluid intake reduce performance. Planning for the meals carefully and consulting the nutritional advisor for the best results. A sports nutritionist can advise both amateur and professional athletes on the best diet to follow in order to achieve their specific demands and objectives.

One may be an active adult exercising for health improvement or a competitive athlete. Whatever the case, sports nutrition will play an important role in achieving success. Sports nutrition is all about eating to achieve specific goals. It can help enhance athletic performance, improve exercise recovery, and make reaching desired goals possible.

6
CELEBRATE A WORLD OF FLAVOURS

Dr Shivangi Gupta

(PhD Home Science)

Working as Clinical Dietician

Celebrating flavours from cultures around the world is a delightful way to nourish ourselves and appreciate our diversity. We are all unique in terms of our body type, goals, lifestyle, culture, tradition and tastes. Trying foods and recipes from various cultures is one fruitful way to include different flavours into our healthy eating routine. Many cuisines offer dishes which include foods from each food group, which makes it possible to plan meals that are nutritious, well-balanced, and are bursting with flavour.

Trying new flavours and foods from around the world can also help one to increase the variety in the foods we eat. Choosing a variety of nutritious foods from all the food groups (cereals, millets and pulses; vegetables and fruits; oils, fats and nuts; and milk and animal foods) in the recommended amounts will help in getting the nutrients that are needed for maintaining a good health.

There are many ways to experiment with global cuisine. Here are some ideas to introduce a whole new range of authentic flavours and foods when planning the meals.

1. Introduce New Cuisines in your Meals

One can start planning their weekly menu by introducing new cuisines in their meal plan such as Mediterranean, Italian, Japanese; Spanish and so on according to one's personal liking and preferences. This will not just help you to explore new textures and flavours but would also make your meal more appealing and interesting.

Another way to explore different cuisines is to try a familiar ingredient in a new way. For Example: - In North India, plain rice is usually served with dal, beans or vegetable curry. One can try making different varieties of rice such as coconut rice, lemon rice, tamarind rice and try it with sambhar, fish/chicken curry, rasam, stuffed bell peppers, mushroom risotto etc.

2. Discover New Flavours with Herbs and Spices

Cooking with different herbs and spices is essential for adding flavour from around the world. Different cuisines use different herbs and spices that are unique to their culture, tradition and geographical area. Addition of these herbs and spices not only will add new taste and aroma to the dish but will also enhance its overall flavour.

3. Try New Fruits and Vegetables

Take the opportunity to explore less familiar fruits and vegetables around you. One can plan a trip to a local/cultural or international food market to discover new varieties of the same. Try to know about their origin, appearance, taste, aroma and other aspects. Including new fruits and vegetables can add variety in our diet and make our meals more enjoyable.

4. Involve Kids and other Family Members in Meal Prepration

Getting kids involved in kitchen helps to expose them to new foods, flavours and ingredients. Choosing meals from new cuisines includes trying new foods together with your loved ones. Get input from the rest of the family to see what new foods or dishes they may want to try and then take some time to prepare it together.

Here is a list of some meals and snacks that can add variety and flavours from around the world:-

• Raw veggies with hummus, which is a creamy yogurt-based dressing made with cucumbers, garlic, and dill.

• Vegetables like cabbage, eggplant, or zucchini can be stuffed with seasoned mixtures that may include meats, grains, and sauces.

• Salads that include different types of produce along with whole grains, dairy, and protein, such as a tuna salad made with Greek yogurt, onion, celery, and whole wheat pasta.

• A Spanish omelette with potatoes and other veggies, topped with a sprinkle of cheese and paprika.

• A smoothie with low-fat yogurt or buttermilk, and tropical fruits like papaya or mango.

On a large scale, food is an important part of our culture, tradition and heritage and an expression of our cultural identity. So, let's celebrate National Nutrition Month by celebrating a world of flavours!

7

FLAVORS OF RAMADAN

Taskeen Fatima

Assistant Professor

St. Joseph's College for Women, Civil Lines, Gorakhpur

Email: taskeen.fatima0101@gmail.com

The month of Ramadan is a time for both religious and non-religiously observant Muslims. Eid al-Fitr marks the end of the fasting month of Ramadan. While Ramadan is an important month in the Islamic calendar and culture, this resources concentrates are three essential parts of Ramadan, which are, in Arabic:

- *Sawm*, or fasting

- *Suhoor* , or starting the fast

- *Iftar*, or breaking the fast on a daily basis

- *Eid al Fitr*, or the end of Ramadan three day feast

Together, these parts of Ramadan provide a good introduction to the month.

Ramadan

The fasting month of Ramadan is the most important month for, Ramadan is the name of the ninth month in the Islamic lunar calendar. The lunar calendar is based on the moon's orbit of the earth of 29 ½ days. Twelve lunar months make a lunar year, which is 354 days long, the lunar year is approximately 11 days shorter than the solar year. In this month Muslims fasts from dawn to dusk.

Ramadan Fasting and the body

During fasting hours when no food or drink is consumed, the body uses its stored carbohydrate (stored in the liver and muscles) and fat to provide energy .As the Ramadan fast only lasts from dawn till dusk, the body's energy can be replaced in the pre-dawn and dusk meals. This provides a gentle transition from using glucose as the main source of energy, to using fat, and prevents the breakdown of muscle for protein. After a few days of the fast, higher levels of endorphins appear in the blood, making one more alert and giving an overall feeling of general mental wellbeing.

Although body cannot store water and hence the kidneys conserve as much water as possible by reducing the amount lost in urine. However, the body cannot avoid losing some water when one goes to the toilet, excrete/sweat through the skin and when someone breathe or when we sweat if it is warm. Depending on the weather and the length of the fast, most people who fast during Ramadan will experience mild dehydration, which may cause headaches, tiredness and difficulty concentrating. If some one is unable to stand up due to dizziness, or individual feel disoriented, they should urgently drink regular, moderate quantities of water – ideally with sugar and salt – a sugary drink or rehydration solution. Once the fast is broken, the body can rehydrate and gain energy from the foods and drinks consumed. Having not eaten for a long period, one may find it helpful to eat slowly after breaking the fast and can be started with plenty of fluids and low-fat, fluid-rich foods.

Effect of fasting on health

Results from studies on the health effects of Ramadan fasting are mixed, probably because the length of the fast and the weather conditions experienced vary depending on the time of year and the country where the fast is being observed. Some studies have found that people lose weight during Ramadan (although they tended to put this weight back on after Ramadan). Few studies have looked at the effect of Ramadan fasting on factors like blood cholesterol and triglycerides (fat in the blood) and found a short term improvement in some cases though some studies found no effect. There have also been some small studies that suggest that Ramadan fasting may have a short term beneficial effect on the immune system. In both cases, the results of studies have been mixed and so more research is needed to confirm these results.

Traditionally there is an emphasis on providing bountiful meal to celebrate this special month. The women of the house toil for hours preparing scrumptious meals for family and friends. Few recipes which are commonly made during Ramadan are Sheer khurma, Zarda, Phirni, Qimami Sewai, shahi tukda, khajoor ka halwa, Seekh kabab, etc.

1. Sheer Khurma (Sewaiya Kheer)

Sheer Khurma is a rich vermicelli pudding, packed with sugary milk, dates and crunchy nuts. Eid festivities are incomplete without a luscious bowl of Sheer Khurma, it is considered to be an auspicious dish to start the holy day.

This delicious Mughlai dessert is a treat for all senses. With the ingredients milk, vermicelli, dates, nuts, saffron, ghee. Milk is rich in calcium content which is good for strengthening of bones, teeth and muscles. Vermicelli is made from wheat flour. It is low in sodium.

High amounts of sodium in blood can increase the risk of high blood pressure. Simultaneously, vermicelli is low in cholesterol and fat as well. Dates are low in fat content and can help in regulating cholesterol levels in the body. They are rich in proteins and vitamins like B Vitamins, Vitamin A and Vitamin C. Dates can help in preventing osteoporosis as they contain high amounts of magnesium, manganese and copper. One can also add cashews to your sheer khurma. Cashews are packed with Vitamins E, Vitamin K and Vitamin B6 along with minerals like copper, phosphorus, magnesium, zinc and iron. Eating nuts like cashews can help lower the risk for cardiovascular diseases and maintain the immune system.

2. Zarda

This sweet rice preparation is a special festive dish relished by Muslims on the occasion of Eid. The name is derived from the Persian word "Zard" which translates to yellow. Full of aromatic spices and laden with mava, ghee and nuts.

Nuts are a nutritionally rich food, containing most of the vitamins and minerals the body needs. They're one of the main sources of omega-3 fatty acids, offering a range of health benefits from reducing rheumatoid arthritis to protecting against Alzheimer's and dementia.

3. Phirni

Phirni hailed from ancient Persia or Middle East and it's the Mughals who both invented and introduced it to India. The Mughal Empire relished the regal milk-based dish and made it popular. It is a healthy, milk based dish. Rice gives nutritional value to the dish and nuts are full of vitamins, proteins and minerals. Only the sugar is the villain here. Diabetic patients and obese people need to be careful.

4. Qimami Sewai

Qimami sewai aka Kimami sewaiyan is one of the most popular classic desserts in the subcontinents of Asia. It is a traditional dessert which is also considered as the heart of Eid festival. This Eid ki seviyan is rich, fragrant, utterly scrumptious and easy to make. In this preparation, ghee roasted vermicelli aka sewai is cooked in flavoured sweet syrup with mawa and lots of dry fruits. It can be served as a dessert after meal or simply as a sweet snack. The word 'kimami' means 'sweet and fragrant' and 'sewai' means 'vermicelli'. It is also popular as eid ki meethi seviyan and dry seviyan etc. It contains vermicelli, mawa, milk, sugar, ghee and lots of dry fruits. As it contain milk and Mawa, they are rich in protein.

High in calcium. Good for bone health and for muscle development. Dry fruits Boosts immunity, helps to lose weight, keeps skin healthy and wrinkle-free, fight against constipation, helps to prevent cancer, maintain a healthy heart. It is also a calorie-dense and fat-rich food. Despite its health benefits, consuming too much ghee can lead to increased weight gain and elevate the risk of obesity.

5. Shahi Tukda

Shahi Tukda is a royal, festive dessert that is made with ghee, bread, sweetened milk and nuts. It is a piece of crisp fried golden colored bread that is topped with some sweetened condensed milk (rabdi) and nuts. The bread is soft yet crispy and has absorbed desi ghee. The flavours of sugar syrup, rabdi and saffron get absorbed by the bread, which makes it taste like a bread pudding. This recipe provides calcium and Vitamin A

6. Khajoor Ka Halwa

Khajoor Ka Halwa is a famous Arabian dessert. This easy recipe is for all the dessert lovers. It is a combination of dates, pistachios, almonds, cardamom, sugar/jaggery and is topped with raisins. Dates are high in fiber and very nutritious and on the other hand jaggery are rich in iron, calcium, magnesium, phosphorus, potassium, sodium, selenium and many more nutritional values

7. Seekh Kabab

Mutton Seekh Kebab is a Mughlai delicacy prepared with minced mutton, onions and a blend of spices. These succulent kebabs are delicious and mildly spicy dish that has incredible taste and flavours. This savory and flavorful recipe provides a nutritionally diverse boost of protein and calcium to meal. Goat meat helps with iron recovery among women during menstruation and provides relief from menstrual pain. .Due to its high content of Vitamin B12, it helps to get healthy skin. And as it is rich omega-3 fatty acids, which is an effective antioxidant .Vitamin B12, helps to beat stress and depression.

Conclusion

Due to presence of various flavorful delicacies, it has been reported that there is indulgence in dietary behaviors that do not meet daily dietary recommendations The quality of foods eaten and eating patterns in Ramadan may be different from other months of the year. This affects different aspects of human health. Researches prove that the effect of fasting on human health produces mixed findings regarding body weight and important nutrient changes. This could lead to a possible trigger of eating disorders during Ramadan. Adequate nutrients and energy intake is therefore critical to growth and development during this one month phase of life.

References

1. Trepanowski JF, Bloomer RJ. The impact of religious fasting on human health. Nutr J. 2010;9:57.
2. Nematy M, Alinezhad-Namaghi M, Rashed MM, Mozhdehifard M, Sajjadi SS, Akhlaghi S, Sabery M, Mohajeri SAR, Shalaey N, Moohebati M, et al. Effects of Ramadan fasting on cardiovascular risk factors: a prospective observational study. Nutr J. 2012;11:6
3. Leiper J, Molla A. Effects on health of fluid restriction during fasting in Ramadan. Eur J ClinNutr. 2003;57:S30–
4. Al-Hourani H, Atoum M. Body composition, nutrient intake and physical activity patterns in young women during Ramadan. Singap Med J. 2007; 48(10):906.

5. Azizi F. Islamic fasting and health. Ann NutrMetab. 2010;56(4):273–82.

6. Toda M, Morimoto K. Effects of Ramadan fasting on the health of Muslims. Nihon eiseigakuzasshi Japanese j hygiene. 2000;54(4):592–6.

7. Poh B, Zawiah H, Ismail M, Henry C. Changes in body weight, dietary intake and activity pattern of adolescents during Ramadan. Malays J Nutr. 1996; 2(1):1–10.

8
FRUITS FOR A HEALTHY LIFE

Dr. Devdatta Lad

Department of Zoology

Wilson College

Chowpatty, Mumbai

A healthy mind lives in a healthy body, as was quoted long ago. But for a healthy body, a balanced diet is a must. In our balanced diet, fruits are a must. Every fruit has unique qualities and biochemical composition that provide nutrition to the body.

This essay highlights some of the important fruits, their biochemical composition and clinical significance. These fruits are easily available in our local markets. Apples contain soluble and insoluble fibre along with pectin, hemicellulose, cellulose, vitamin C, and polyphenol. Apples promote good digestion, immunity, and lower the risk of heart disease, obesity, stroke, cancer, and certain neurological disorders. Bananas contain potassium, vitamin C, vitamin B6, magnesium, polyphenols, and polysterols. Bananas promote the growth of beneficial bacteria in the gut. They are an excellent source of dietary fibre, which improves digestive health, and they are known as an instant source of energy food. Vitamin C, potassium, folate, thiamine (B1), fiber, and polyphenols are all found in oranges and sweet limes. Oranges and sweet lime lower the levels of inflammation, blood pressure, cholesterol, and post-meal blood sugar. Oranges and sweet limes are a high source of antioxidants.

Mangoes are a rich source of potassium, folate, fibre, vitamin A, C, B6, E, and K, polyphenols, and antioxidants. Mangoes improve digestive health by increasing bowel movement. Mangoes protect our bodies from chronic diseases such as Type 2 diabetes, heart diseases, Alzheimer's, Parkinson's, and cancer. Pineapple is high in vitamin C, manganese, polyphenolic compounds, and the enzyme bromelain. Pineapple supports metabolism and blood sugar regulation. It has antioxidant and anti-inflammatory properties. It supports digestion. Strawberries reduce the risk of chronic disease as they contain Vitamin C, folate, manganese, polyphenols, flavonoids, phenolic acids, lignans, tannins, anthocyanins, ellagitannins, and proanthocyanidins.

Watermelon contains vitamins A, C, Beta-carotene, lycopene, potassium, and magnesium. All this matter in watermelon lowers levels of oxidative stress and inflammation, and also decreases the risk of cancer, heart diseases, and type 2 diabetes, provides skin protection by helping skin heal faster, helps hydrate and replenish electrolytes in the body. Kiwi fruit is loaded with Vitamin C, dietary fiber, potassium, folate, Vitamin E, carotenoids, lutein, zeaxanthin, beta carotene, polyphenols, and the enzyme actinidin. This content of Kiwi supports eye health, gut health, and digestion by softening stools and treating mild constipation. Peaches contain potassium, dietary fiber, Vitamin A, C, and E, lutein, zeaxanthin, and beta-carotene. These assist in fighting free radicals in the body. Guava is a common Indian fruit that possesses vitamins, lycopene, and Beta Carotene. All these support the good health of the eyes, heart, kidney, skin, and increase immunity. Grapes are fortified with potassium, vitamin K, resveratrol, anthocyanins, caffeic acid, quercetin, and kaempferol. This supports heart and brain health and also reduces the risk of certain types of cancer. Pomegranates possess antioxidants and anti-inflammatory properties. They also reduce the risk of certain chronic diseases. This is due to the presence of flavonoids, tannins, and lignans.

Jackfruits are known to improve vision, cure anaemia, prevent cardio-vascular diseases, blood pressure, and diabetes, support bone health, aid digestion, and weight loss. Jackfruit is laden with Vitamin A, C, and E, Beta-Carotene, copper, manganese, magnesium, potassium, and resveratrol. Jamun keeps the blood sugar level low. It has astringent properties as it protects the skin from pimples, wrinkles, and acne. It boosts haemoglobin production. It has fructose, Vitamin C, calcium, phosphorus, sodium, potassium, magnesium, thiamine, riboflavin, carotene, folic acid, and dietary fibres. Vitamin C, Vitamin B1 (Thiamine). Potassium, catechin, epicatechin and epigallacatechin are present in custard apple. Thus, the custard apple promotes eye health, prevents high blood pressure and inflammation, improves digestion, immunity, and has anticancer properties. Thus, fruits are important for a healthy life.

9

IMPORTANCE OF MICRONUTRIENTS FOR COGNITIVE FUNCTIONS IN DAILY LIFE

Neelam

Research Scholar

Department of Home Science

Mahila Mahavidyalaya, Banaras Hindu University, Varanasi

Email: neelampaswan@bhu.ac.in,

"Yatha Annam Tatha Mannam"

(Mental and intellectual development is directly related to the quality of our food intake)

Micronutrients are essential for maintaining tissue function and metabolism in daily life. Vitamins and minerals are the nutrients that the body needs in extremely small amounts. However, they have a crucial impact on one's holistic health, and a lack of any one of them can lead to serious, even life-threatening illnesses. They carry out a variety of tasks, including assisting the body in producing the hormones, enzymes, and other elements necessary for growth and development. The most prevalent nutritional deficiencies worldwide, particularly in children and pregnant women, are those due to iron, vitamin A, and iodine. Micronutrient deficiencies are disproportionately prevalent in low- and middle-income counties. These deficiencies have been attributed to age-related cognitive decline and therefore can affect cognitive function at any stage of life. Micronutrient supplementation can help persons to reduce the risk of deficiencies prevalent among them, which may help maintain cognitive function. The four basic groups of micronutrients, vitamins, and minerals include water-soluble vitamins, fat-soluble vitamins, macro minerals, and trace minerals.

Vitamin A, Vitamin B Complex, and Vitamin C

Vitamin A (Retinol) affects the brain. The retinoid regulate neuronal differentiation, and they may also play a role in memory, sleep, depression, Parkinson's disease, and Alzheimer's disease. Moreover, the formation of neuronal myelin sheet and the proper functioning of the brain all depend on vitamin B_{12} because impaired cognitive development is connected to inadequate vitamin B_{12} status among children and other negative effects on a child's health. Therefore, vitamin B_{12} is crucial for neural myelination, synaptogenesis, and neurotransmitter production all of which have an impact on how the brain develops and functions. Ascorbic acid known as Vitamin C is an antioxidant. It participates in neuronal maturation, myelination, and neurotransmitter-mediated cell signalling in the central nervous system. Also essential as an antioxidant in the brain because a sufficient supply of Ascorbic acid is required to avoid damage from oxidative stress since neurons are particularly susceptible to it. Vitamin B complex (Riboflavin, Pyridoxine, Cyanocobalamin, nicotinamide, folate) and Ascorbic acid are specifically required for the metabolism of dopamine and noradrenaline within the CNS.

Omega 3, Zinc, Iron and Iodine

Omega 3 (Polyunsaturated fatty acids) are important for the development of the children's brains because, they play a substantial role in neurogenesis, neurotransmission, and neuroprotection. Zinc is an essential micro mineral that is containing 200 enzymes and many proteins, hormones, hormone receptors, and neuropeptides also require zinc as a structural component. While the precise function of zinc in the brain is still unknown, It has been shown that one of the main health consequences of zinc shortage is cognitive impairment. Iron is a co-factor for several enzymes involved in the manufacture of neurotransmitters, including tryptophan hydroxylase (serotonin) and tyrosine hydroxylase (norepinephrine and dopamine). Iron also impacts the correct myelination of neurons. Iodine is another an essential mineral for the production of the thyroid hormones triiodothyronine (T_3) and thyroxine (T_4), both of which are necessary for the growth and development of the brain or cognitive development.

Calcium and Magnesium

Calcium plays a crucial role in the regulation of neurotransmission, intracellular communication, and neuronal excitability. Intake of calcium and magnesium according to RDA 2020 is 1000mg/day and 270-320mg/day. More than 300 enzymes depend on magnesium for proper function, and it also helps regulate neuro chemical transmission and muscle excitability.

Source of Micronutrients

Micronutrients are an essential element for cognitive development. Therefore, the daily should include fruits and vegetables, milk and milk products in the plate. According to RDA 400 g/day of fruits and vegetables should include in diet with the purpose of obtaining enough antioxidant nutrients such as beta-carotene, vitamin C and certain non-nutrients like polyphenols and flavonoids which may protect against chronic diseases.

Rainbow Diet

The Rainbow Diet was first created in 2005 as a fusion between the colourful Mediterranean Diet and the French Paradox by former Oxford University Biochemist, Chris Woollams, who developed a cutting-edge approach to the benefits of good versus bad fats, whole grains, sugar, and colourful fruits and vegetables, updating frequently as new studies consistently demonstrated the numerous health benefits of bioactive substances.

Hence, Micronutrients plays and important role for cognitive functions in daily life. Not only helps in maintaining brain function but also maintains the growth and development of the individual. Fruits, vegetables, and dairy products are the best sources of these nutrients and should all be included in the daily diet.

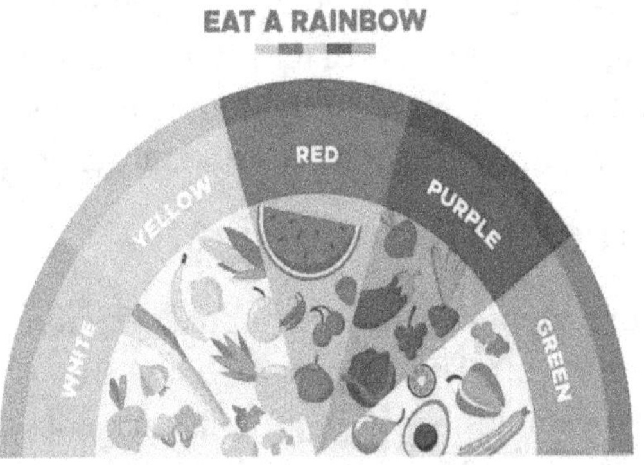

Keeping oneself physically fit is just not sufficient to live a healthier and comfortable life but one needs to have a healthy body with a healthy mind.

10

MY PERSONAL JOURNEY - NUTRITION IN BED BOUND PATIENTS

Dr. Shweta Habbu Acharya

Reader, Dept. of Public Health Dentistry,

Dr. HSRSM Dental College and Hospital, Hingoli

It was 6th October 2021, the worst hit us. My husband suffered from a massive brain stroke, the stroke which had prevalence of only 2% among such cases. It shook my entire family, and we were completely unaware of what we are going to face in the due course of time. It was indeed the worst time of our lives, with doctors telling us to be prepared for more than the worst... And when after 45 days of struggle, he was out of ventilator; doctors exclaimed that it was not less than a miracle! We lived it through it all...

Then the neuro-physician suggested another procedure to make his nutrition better by inserting a tube directly into the stomach. But having another surgery after him having pipes through most of his organs- tracheostomy tube, extra-ventricular drain, urinary catheter; we were not mentally prepared at all. Being a doctor, I knew that only two things, beyond the divine blessings of course, were going to help in his long and exhausting recovery; and they were the physiotherapy and good nutrition. So, we went for the procedure... and we got the Percutaneous Endoscopic Gastrostomy (PEG) tube inserted.

We started the journey towards his recovery with the PEG tube, which was completely new to us, and later came to know that it was not only new to us, but the hospital nurses, dietician, and most of the doctors also. Every new nurse had to be informed, most of them had only followed the protocol of the nasogastric tube before. I read a lot on the internet, but sadly nothing useful or related was available. We searched for recipes we could give him but no Indian recipes were available, so we ended up giving him liquids only. I was sad that we went for an entire procedure only to improve his nutrition and we are giving him what we could give through nasogastric tube. It was all in vain. Why did he and we have to go through all this!

As we got him home, we took up courage and started experimenting with food that we could give. We had no one to guide us what to give him or how to keep the tube clean, what to do if it was blocked, what to do if it came out. It even did come out one day. And we rushed to the hospital. The doctors relieved us saying rather it took time with you, the tube comes out earlier than this in other patients and we don't need to worry. Still, we had to spend five days at hospital due to the unavailability of the tube in a tier 2 city.

And after months of trying to find some more information and contemplation we discovered that we could give him the exact same food by semi-solidifying the same the rest of us eat at home. The semi-solid, increased the density and variety of food. Him being a big time foodie, we missed giving him so many things which he liked, all because no one was aware of this method of feeding.

This is the condition of awareness and support in case of the nutrition in bed bound patients. A lot of research papers, all foreign, lots of recipes, but all non-vegetarian and using products which are probably not available here, so we really had a tough time figuring out how to give and what to give. Now we feel guilty for giving him only liquids when we could had given him a better nutrition. The availability, awareness and support for nutrition in the bed bound patients' needs to take into serious considerations by medical and nutrition community to reduce the sufferings of patients and their families. More awareness among community and medical fraternity need to be done with special focus on Indian population.

11

FLAVOURS OF BENGAL

Aishwarya Das

Research scholar

Department of Home Science (Foods and Nutrition)

Mahila Mahavidyalaya, Banaras Hindu University

Varanasi

Email: taishwarya2025@gmail.com

West Bengal is a state in the eastern part of India along with Bay of Bengal with 91 million inhabitants. Kolkata is the capital as well as heart of the Bengal. The kitchen of every Bengalis must contain a variety of flavourful ingredients like panch phoron (five spices),shorshe tel(mustard oil), kalo jeera (nigella seeds),posto (poppy seeds), Shorshe posto powder (mustard seed and poppy seed powder). Bengalis are all about good food, with their distinct cooking methods and ingredients that are low on spice and oil and the foods are simply die for. Before going to the details cooking process of some special dishes by bengalis and nutritive value of them, a little bit addition about mentioned flavourful ingredients are discussed.

Panch phoron

It is the mixture of five spices in seed form – fenugreek, black mustard, nigella, cumin and fennel. It is the basic essence of bengali kitchen and the power to enhance the taste of any dish without need to add any other flavours to it.

Sorshe tel

Bengalis prefer to cook with mustard oil over refined oil, be it vegetarian or non vegetarian dishes. Its pungent aroma is very much preferred by the bengalis. Besides providing this unique aroma mustard oil contains Omega-3 and Omega-6 fatty acids which lowers the risk associated with heart diseases.

Kalo jeera

Basically kalonji or nigella seeds dominate aroma and flavours of traditional bengali dishes. This ingredient in combination with mustard oil and dry chilles or shukno lanka   creates the magic.

Posto

The royalty or richness of every bengali dish is maintained addition of posto or poppy seeds in form of aloo posto means potato in poppy seed. If a soul food had a face, it would be posto or poppy seed. Some of the famous and rich dishes of Bengal and their nutritional concern are highlighted below:

Shorshe Ilish Bhapa

This is a traditional and typical Bengali dish known as steamed hilsa prepared by bengalis using Hilsa fish (Ilish Mach) and the secret of its identical pungent flavour is just because of the presence of paste of ground mustard powder. A few whole green chilli, turmeric and common salt are used to prepare the dish. Hilsa has a triglyceride (TG) lowering effect and hence beneficial for reducing the risk of heart diseases. This also provides a good amount of protein also. As frying is not needed do not cause any gastrointestinal irritation. This also provides a good amount of sodium.

Shukto

This one is another kind of famous dish only made by Bengalis. This dish is basically a mixture of atleast nine vegetable including potato, bingal, raw banana, papaya, bitterguard, sweet potato and moringa sticks. This is typically known as navaratna curry in other state but the basic difference is in the flavour is that bengalis makes it bitter and slightly sweet in taste and use of Panch phoron is the main secret behind this traditional dish. Mustard oil, milk, ghee, turmeric and salts are also used to prepare. This generally served with rice. The tradition of starting meal with bitters, considered to have a medicinal value and anciently suggested by authors of ayurveda. Shukto was consumed as a cooling food agent in the hot and humid climates of the ancient kingdom of undivided bengal like Anga, Vanga, and Kalinga, Moreover due the vegetable content it provides a good amounts of micronutrients.

Aloo posto

Another typical Bengali preparation is aloo posto that is potato in poppy seeds. Every Bengali likes to have aloo posto in their thali during summer days this because it is beleived to cool the stomach during hot humid weather. Besides this poppy seeds contain vitamin B complex, fibre, calcium, magnesium and zinc which are essential to meet the nutritional needs of the body.

Here some of the common and typical traditional flavouful ingredients and receips using them are discussed. But Bengal is also famous for using Misti Doi (sweet curd) and rasogolla as sweet dish after their meals. Several variants of these traditional dishes are now becoming available in the restaurants but secrets of typical bengali flavours always remains behind the kitchens of home of every Bengali.

12

INDIAN SPICES: FLAVOURS OF WORLD & FLAVOURS IN HEALTH

Ranjana Sinha,

Research Scholar,

P.G. Department of Home Science,

Magadh University, Bodhgaya

Aroma is a qualitative element and a crucial part of flavour. Flavours are a complex amalgamation of several substances that are either isolated from their original forms in natural sources like plants or animals or created artificially in a lab. Natural flavouring substances are created from essential nutrients like lipids and amino acids. Subconsciously, we rely on taste and scent to find nutrient-rich food. Our cuisine has changed drastically recently, and the flavour is no longer what it always was.

In order to preserve our health and meet our nutritional needs, flavour is crucial. It is believed that a certain centre in our brain causes cravings pertinent to alleviate deficiencies of proven excesses based on the natural nutritional profile of an individual. As a result of sensory exposure to the product or its flavour, these cravings develop. Thus, flavourings in food and products help people achieve physiologically optimal nutrition.The flavour of spices has a significant impact on how Indians prepare and eat food. Due to their rich and spicy flavours, Indian curries are adored worldwide. Each spice has a distinct flavour and aroma. However, the advantages of Indian spices go beyond flavour and taste. Indian spices enhance the flavour of the cuisine. However, scientists from all around the world have examined the health advantages of Indian spices and come up with commendable findings For instance, golden milk (turmeric milk) has become extremely popular throughout the world as a great immunity booster, especially during the current pandemic. Fortunately, since turmeric is a crucial component of Indian food, we have been eating it from childhood in India.

Indian spices, used in everything from cooking to medicine, have long been an important part of Indian cuisine. Spices are used to flavour, colour, and preserve food in addition to improving palatability. Over 100 common spices are used in cuisine all over the world, and they are rich sources of antioxidants Given how flavorful the spices are, it is simpler to utilise less unhealthy ingredients like salt, sugar, and added fat. But not all spices are equally beneficial to the body or effective. Numerous Indian spices enhance the nutritious value of food while also giving it a distinctive flavour. Here are some Indian spices that will nourish and energise you.

Turmeric

Turmeric contains bioactive substances with potent therapeutic effects. The primary active component of turmeric, cur cumin, has potent anti-inflammatory properties and is a potent antioxidant. Therefore, ingesting turmeric has a variety of advantages, such as improving immunity, lowering cholesterol, preventing cancer, and alleviating arthritis symptoms. The AYUSH MANTRALAYA became aware of the "GOLDEN MILK" pandemic. During this pandemic, golden milk became highly famous.

Cinnamon

It is also known as "dalchini." It is a well-liked spice that may be utilised in a variety of dishes and baked goods. Cinnamon has demonstrated antioxidant qualities that can help combat inflammation. By slowing down the digestion of carbs and enhancing insulin sensitivity, it can lower blood sugar levels. Cinnamaldehyde, a substance in cinnamon, is responsible for its therapeutic effects. The recommended daily intake of cinnamon is between 1 and 6 grammes; higher quantities may be hazardous.

Fenugreek

Studies have shown that fenugreek seeds, also known as methi seeds, can lower blood sugar, increase a mother's ability to produce breast milk, reduce calorie intake and appetite, lessen heartburn, improve metabolism, and manage diabetes. Fenugreek is typically safe for healthy persons and does not appear to have any adverse effects.

Cumin seeds

Cumin has high iron content by nature and may aid in weight loss. According to studies, black cumin is particularly efficient against "various infectious diseases owing to bacterial, fungal, parasitic, and viral infections" as well as "neurological and mental sickness, cardiovascular disorders, cancer, diabetes, inflammatory conditions, and infertility." It possesses anti-cancerous qualities. Everyday use of cumin seeds in food helps strengthen the body's defences against a number of chronic illnesses.

Black pepper

Due to its ability to purify the body, black pepper is sometimes referred to as the "KING OF SPICES" and helps with weight loss and improved digestion. Black pepper has anti-inflammatory, anti-asthmatic, anti-fungal, anti-amoebic, and antioxidant properties. It contains "PIPERINE," a bioactive substance. From black pepper to saffron, these spices have enhanced the flavour of already-flavoured culinary items while also providing health advantages.

Conclusion

In addition to providing nutritious flavour, Indian spices have health advantages that help the body fight off free radicals and build immunity. Of fact, not all of the health benefits of Indian spices have been established, but since they are still a vital component of Indian cooking, moderate consumption is safe for healthy people. Numerous researches from throughout the world have demonstrated the numerous health benefits of Indian spices.

13
IMPORTANCE OF NUTRITION IN DAILY LIFE

Dr. Purrvi Patel,

Homoeopathic physician, nutritionist, Mindfulness coach for adults and teens, Author.

Introduction

"Nutrition" What kind of thoughts comes in our mind when you read this word "Nutrition"? Did you have thoughts of food or diet or vitamins or minerals or protein or carbohydrate or fats? So, to understand importance of nutrition in daily life first we need to understand:

What is Nutrition?

In simple words Nutrition means studying of nutrients in food, how the body uses them, and the relationship between diet, health and disease.

What does food means to our body?

For body food means certain kinds of macronutrients and micronutrients. Macronutrients has calorific values while micronutrients have zero calorific values. Our body needs energy to perform certain functions like digestion, blood circulation, renal functions, for movements of bones and joints etc. We get this energy from eating food. Find in below figure what are the micronutrients and what are the macronutrients which comprises of any food we eat and it is very important for us to know about them.

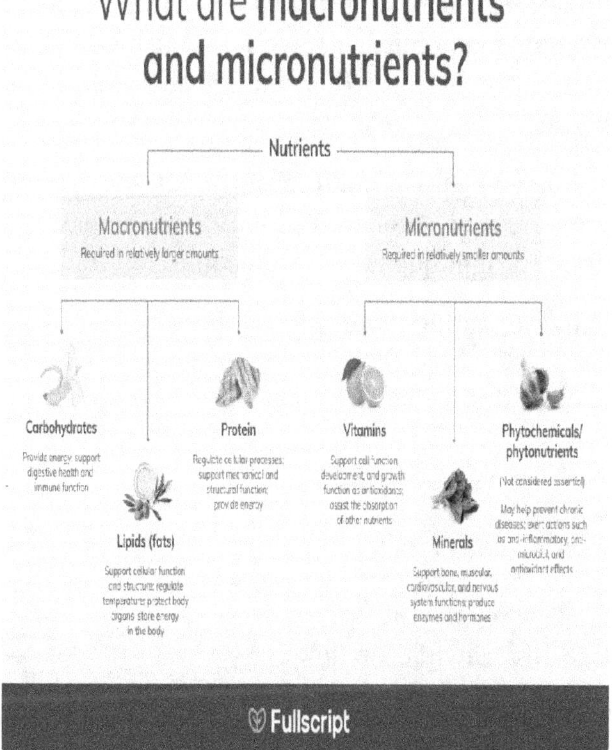

So, to run all these functions of our body we need to eat 1. healthy and balanced food which contain all the micro and macro nutrients in balanced form. Wrong eating pattern, lack of sleep, inadequate amount of water intake and living sedentary life (lack of exercise)invites all kind of lifestyle diseases like Diabetes, Hypertension, Thyroid gland dysfunction, Obesity, PCOS etc.

As per research our plate should contain 50% of salads,

25% ofprotein,15% of carbohydrate and 10% of fats. This means it is very important for us to eat all nutrients to have healthy and fit body as well as mind. Not a single nutrient is bad, bad is the quantities which we sometimes exceed to satiate our taste buds. When we eat more protein and less carb or less fats and more protein it will disturb our metabolism as well as hormonal synthesis which is more harmful then eating all kinds of food at longer run.

So, to have healthy and to ensure that you are eating all nutrients in required quantity follow 4 principals of eating right food in right quantity at right time.

4principals of eating food:

1. Why and when you eat?

2. What you eat?

3. How you eat?

4. How much you eat?

Let's see all4principles in detail:

1. Why and when you eat?

There are 3 kinds of WHY to eatfood

>Need

>want

>Beliefs and rules

Whenever you feel hungry ask yourself is this real hunger or you want to eat due to any temptation. Soon after eating if you feel hungry then it must be thirst and by mistake you feel that you are hungry again or if you have temptation for your favorite sweet after eating then it is yours want of eating not the real hunger. The real hunger is your need to give energy to your body in form of food. When you have to eat only certain kind of food as a part of some rituals or festival fast then also it will disturb your metabolism. You can always choose food wisely in order to follow rituals.

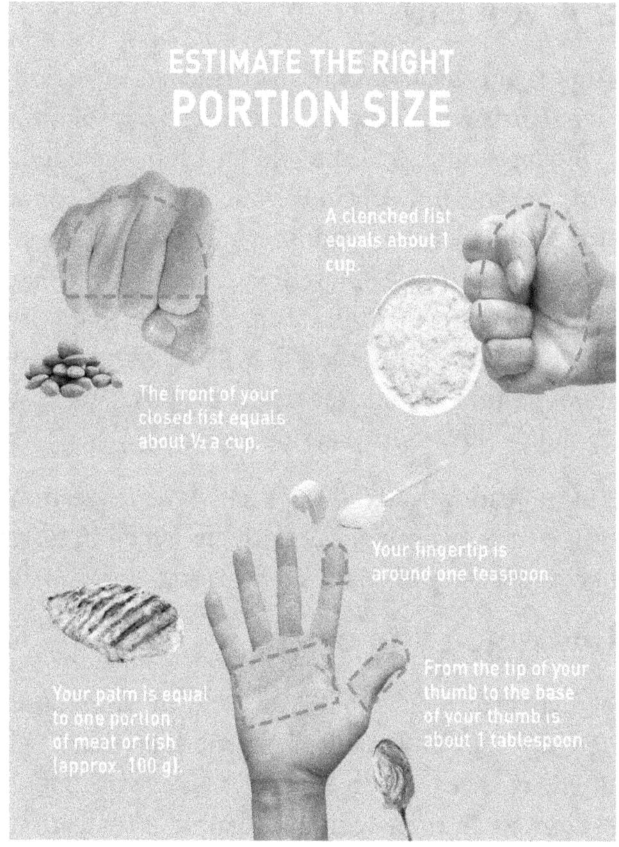

2. What to eat?

We all knows now that we have to eat all the nutrients in balanced quantity. To have all nutrients in balanced form follow the below rules:

>A serving of PROTEIN=Size of your palm

>A serving of CARBOHYDRATE=1 cupped hand size

>A serving of FAT= 1 thumb size

>A serving of VEGGIES AND FRUITS=1 fist size

3. How you eat?

Now this is the most important principal of eating food. You need to be, mindful while eating your food. Notice what you are eating, feel the smell of food, see and touch the food with awareness, chew your food slowly and enjoy your food while eating. Choose your food before you eat and once you choose then be grateful for it and eat mindfully. If you crib after eating the food that why I eat that and why I eat this then it will be more harmful to your body. Don't watch television or check messages on your mobile while you are eating our food.

Mindful eating aids in process of digestion and absorption of nutrient very effectively which in turn helps in reducing bloating and stops overeating.

4. How much you eat?

As per ayurveda you should eat 80% of your hunger to keep space for air and water. This will help you to eat less unwanted calories. Such habits make you feel more energetics rather then feeling lethargic after eating your meal. There should be energy balance.

Calories in v/s Calories out:

- ➢ Eat more, use less=weight gain

- ➢ Eat less, use more =temporary weight loss

- ➢ Eat=Use=weight maintained

So, now when you know what are the nutrients and how much they are important in our life you can follow all these 4 principles to make maximum use of these nutrients and when all the nutrients taken in balanced quantity there are lesser chances for you to have any lifestyle disease.